BULLETPROOF DIET FOR BEGINNERS

The Complete Guide to Easy Weight Loss, Optimal Brain Health, Blood Sugar Control, Improve Gut Health and Increasing Energy Level

John Hendricks

COPYRIGHT PAGE

© 2024 by John Hendricks

Disclaimer: The information provided in this cookbook is for general informational purposes only. It is not intended as a substitute for professional medical advice, diagnosis, or treatment. Always seek the advice of your physician or other qualified health care provider with any questions you may have regarding a medical condition. The author and publisher are not responsible for any adverse effects or consequences resulting from the use of the recipes or information presented in this cookbook.

Table of Contents

INTRODUCTION

Entrepreneur and biohacker Dave Asprey came up with the Bulletproof Diet as a way to eat to maximize mental and physical performance. Based on biohacking concepts, this diet aims to limit or eliminate specific foods while increasing the consumption of healthy fats, proteins, and veggies with minimal toxins. The basic idea is that by carefully choosing foods that nourish the body without triggering inflammation or blood sugar surges, one may improve energy levels, cognitive function, and general health. The Bulletproof Roadmap is a helpful tool for making healthy food choices since it classifies foods into three zones: Green (very beneficial), Yellow (moderate), and Red (best avoided). The Bulletproof way of life is comprehensive in its approach to health and performance; it goes beyond just diet to optimize sleep, manage stress, and implement tailored biohacking techniques. People looking to maximize their physical and mental potential have found this diet to be an attractive option because to its focus on sustained energy, mental clarity, and long-term well-being.

PART ONE: The Bulletproof Diet

The central tenet of the Bulletproof Diet, a dietary strategy promoted by businessman Dave Asprey, is the maximization of mental and physical performance by the use of certain foods. Incorporating nutrient-dense, high-quality meals while limiting pollutants is the diet's core premise. Consuming "Bulletproof" foods—mainly, high-quality fats, proteins, and low-toxin veggies—is crucial, according to Asprey.

Fats are lauded in this nutritional paradigm for the vital role they play in promoting brain function and general well-being, rather than condemned.

Finding good fats like avocados, grass-fed butter, and coconut oil is a big deal on this diet. The same holds true for the need of high-quality proteins for metabolic health and muscle maintenance; they may be found in foods like pastured eggs and grass-fed meats.

Important to the Bulletproof Diet is the Bulletproof Roadmap, which divides foods into three zones: the "Green Zone," where you should eat them without restriction, and the "Yellow Zone," where you should eat them with some care. People can see exactly what to focus when planning their meals each day thanks to this methodical technique. Nutritionally dense meals are promoted in the Green Zone, but items with potentially harmful effects on health should be consumed in moderation or avoided completely in the Yellow and Red Zones, respectively.

The Bulletproof Diet calls for meal plans that include templates for protein, carb, and fat consumption. In order to help you create meals that adhere to the principles of the program, Asprey gives sample meal plans and recipes. Beyond dietary restrictions, the diet also emphasizes the importance of other lifestyle habits, such as getting enough sleep, controlling stress, and using biohacking strategies.

The Bulletproof Diet also includes strategies for overcoming typical obstacles and breaking through fitness plateaus. Along the way, people may face challenges; the diet provides strategies for overcoming them. Testimonials and success stories showing improvements in physical and mental health provide more evidence of the real-world effects of living the Bulletproof way of life.

Beyond its nutritional component, the Bulletproof Diet promotes a more all-encompassing view of health by teaching its adherents to biohack their way to peak performance in other areas of life. Asprey aspires to build a community of people who will improve their health and wellness by making smart decisions, practicing mindfulness, and sticking to the Bulletproof lifestyle.

Principles and Philosophy

Improving cognitive and physical capacities by deliberate food selection is the central tenet of the Bulletproof Diet. The idea that the body may be optimized by utilizing high-quality fats, proteins, and low-toxin veggies is fundamental to this concept. Sustaining energy, mental clarity, and general well-being are all goals of the diet, which promotes nutrient-dense food intake. The Bulletproof Diet promotes biohacking by stressing the significance of self-awareness and the ability to respond appropriately to one's physiological needs.

The fundamental principle of the diet is to use healthy fats as an energy source, which are abundant in foods like avocados, grass-fed butter, and coconut oil. We think these fats help keep our hormones in check, our cells strong, and our brains working properly. In order to maintain normal muscle function and regeneration, the diet also stresses the need of eating high-quality proteins, such as eggs from pastured animals and grass-fed meats.

With its color-coded "Green," "Yellow," and "Red" zones, the Bulletproof Roadmap provides a useful foundation for the diet. By providing a methodical framework, this method helps people strike a better balance between nourishing their bodies and avoiding harmful substances. By adhering to this plan, followers hope to get metabolic flexibility, which will enable their bodies to burn carbs and fats for fuel more effectively.

The ideas of the Bulletproof Diet go beyond just diet and into other areas of lifestyle choice, such as stress management, getting enough sleep, and developing one's own unique biohacking arsenal. The diet takes a more holistic view of health, viewing the body as an adaptive system that can be fine-tuned by making smart decisions about food as well as other lifestyle elements like exercise, mindfulness, and sleep hygiene.

To boil it down, the Bulletproof food is more than simply a food plan; it's an entire philosophy of life that promotes optimum living and biohacking as a means to help people take charge of their own health and performance.

Understanding Your Body and Energy

Starting the Bulletproof Diet is more than just changing your food habits; it's an in-depth investigation into how your body works and how to tap into its power. The Bulletproof Diet is essentially more than just tracking calories; it takes a more comprehensive approach. It explores the complexities of how various diets impact your vitality, brainpower, and health in general.

Understanding the importance of good fats as a fuel source is a fundamental tenet of the Bulletproof Diet. Healthy fats are really your body's best friends when it comes to providing long-term energy, contrary to popular belief. Ingredients like avocado, coconut oil, and grass-fed butter transform into vital fuel sources that help you stay energized all day long.

Finding the sweet spot for your energy levels requires knowledge of how your body reacts to various meals. The Bulletproof Diet stresses the need of monitoring one's biofeedback, or the how one's body responds to certain diets. By using this individualized approach, you may learn which foods may be contributing to inflammation or energy dumps, and then adjust your diet accordingly.

Energy is a mental as well as a physical concept. Understanding the interdependence between mind and body is central to the Bulletproof Diet. The goal of the diet is to improve energy and productivity by enhancing mental clarity and attention through the consumption of nutrient-dense meals and the incorporation of brain-boosting ingredients such as Bulletproof Coffee.

Also, the Bulletproof Diet stresses the need of knowing that energy demands come and go in cycles. Cyclical ketosis is based on the idea of purposefully alternating periods of high-carb and low-carb eating to force the body to use fat for energy. Not only does this help with weight control, but it also educates your body to use its energy resources more efficiently.

The Bulletproof Diet is essentially an investigation into one's own nature, with an emphasis on learning one's physiological responses rather than merely controlling one's food intake. The key is to incorporate excellent fats into your diet, pay attention to your biofeedback signals, understand the mind-body link, and use energy in cycles. By gaining this all-encompassing knowledge, you give yourself the power to make decisions that fuel your body and allow it to reach its maximum potential.

Biohacking and Body Awareness

Starting the Bulletproof Diet isn't only about changing your food; it's about delving into biohacking and becoming more self-aware. Within the framework of this diet, biohacking takes on a more individual meaning as people search for methods to improve their health and performance. It's all about discovering one's maximum mental and physical potential via scientific inquiry and personal experimentation.

Biohacking on the Bulletproof Diet is around paying close attention to the caliber of the food you provide your body. It's not only about watching calorie intake; it's about selecting foods that are potent partners in the pursuit of peak performance. Recognizing the importance of high-quality fats for sustained energy and general health, the diet gives them special attention. You can biohack your body's energy systems using grass-fed butter, MCT oil, and avocados; they're more than just nutrients.

On the Bulletproof Diet, paying attention to one's body and learning to read its complex signals takes center stage. With the use of biofeedback, people are able to pinpoint which meals may be triggering inflammatory responses, lethargy, or other negative side effects. By being more cognizant, one may customize their approach, turning their nutrition into a living, breathing part of their self-care routine.

Biohacking on the Bulletproof Diet goes beyond what you eat to encompass other aspects of your lifestyle that have an effect on your health. An essential part of this method is the optimization of sleep, the control of stress, and mindful practices. Biohacking is an approach to health and wellness that takes a more holistic view of lifestyle modification in order to improve the body's function by addressing the myriad of elements that affect it.

One of the most prominent biohacking tools is Bulletproof Coffee, which is an integral part of the diet. People can improve their cognitive function and energy levels by mixing grass-fed butter with MCT oil and high-quality coffee. As a biohack, this intentional blend improves concentration and mental clarity while giving you steady energy without the crash that regular coffee usually gives you.

The Bulletproof Diet is, at its core, an adventure in biohacking and increased bodily awareness that leads to greater personal power. By delving into the complex relationships between diet, lifestyle, and performance, it empowers individuals to actively improve their health. Individuals can begin on a revolutionary journey toward reaching peak vitality and unleashing their body's full potential by embracing biohacking ideas and fostering body awareness.

Metabolism and Energy Systems

PART TWO: Bulletproof Foods

The idea of Bulletproof Foods encompasses a method of nutrition that is more than just providing food within the context of the Bulletproof Diet. We choose these foods with an eye toward providing a variety of nutrients that promote peak mental and physical performance, not just calories. The focus is on providing the body with nutritious, high-quality alternatives that are also clean.

When selecting Bulletproof Foods, we looked for those that would boost energy, help with focus, and generally make us feel better. An essential part of the Bulletproof Diet, grass-fed butter is more than just a spread; it's a food supply of healthy fats like omega-3s and CLA, which provide you energy all day long without the crash that regular butter usually causes.

The medium-chain triglyceride (MCT) oil that Bulletproof Foods uses is made from coconuts. This rich supply of medium-chain triglycerides provides a fast and effective way to fuel your body, since it is easily turned into ketones. Not only is it used in cooking, but it also has biohacking properties that improve metabolic health and cognitive performance.

Adding Bulletproof Coffee to your daily routine elevates coffee to a whole new level. People make a combination that has a pleasant flavor, helps with concentration and energy levels all day long by combining high-quality, mold-free coffee beans with grass-fed butter and MCT oil.

Incorporating nutrient-dense proteins like grass-fed meats and wild-caught fish into the Bulletproof Diet guarantees that people get all the protein they need and more, along with other important nutrients like CLA and omega-3 fatty acids. Crucial sources of fiber and a variety of vitamins and minerals, vegetables—especially those low in pollutants and abundant in nutrients—play an important role in a healthy diet.

Avocados, almonds, and extra virgin olive oil are examples of healthy fats that the diet promotes. Not only do these fats make food taste better and make you feel fuller for longer, but they also add to your diet's nutritional profile.

As a whole, Bulletproof Foods are curated with the Bulletproof Diet's guiding principles in mind, which center on a diet rich in healthy fats, lean meats, and nutrient-dense veggies. A more comprehensive view of nutrition takes into account the effects of food on energy, cognition, and health as a whole, rather than focusing solely on macronutrient composition. The Bulletproof Diet is a path to optimal nutrition that aims to help people reach their maximum physical potential via the integration of certain smart dietary choices.

High-Quality Fats

Exploring the world of Bulletproof Diet high-quality fats reveals a nutritional approach that challenges traditional eating habits. Instead than promoting a complete lack of fat, the diet stresses the need of eating good fats on a regular basis. The distinguishing feature of this technique is its fundamental premise, which states that lipids are necessary for general health and vigor.

Beyond just making you feel full, healthy fats have many other advantages. They are essential for maintaining steady energy levels, hormone balance, and brain function. Good fats aren't bad for you; in fact, they're essential for running all of your body's functions. An important part of the Bulletproof diet is eating high-quality fats, which have several beneficial effects, such as improving cognitive function and increasing metabolism.

On the Bulletproof Diet, you may get healthy fats from a wide variety of sources. As a nutritional powerhouse, grass-fed butter shines due to its abundance of omega-3 fatty acids and healthy CLA. Avocados are a flexible complement to meals because of their nutritious richness and monounsaturated fats. Coconut-based medium-chain triglyceride (MCT) oil provides a quick and easily metabolizable energy source, which in turn increases ketone generation.

The heart and inflammation are both helped by the omega-3 fatty acids that are present in fatty fish such as sardines and salmon. Because it contains monounsaturated fats and antioxidants, extra virgin olive oil adds taste to food and salads. For a delicious crunch and a good amount of healthy fats, try nuts and seeds like chia seeds and almonds.

The Bulletproof Diet stresses the importance of choosing good fats over consuming a lot of bad ones. Those following this diet plan may enjoy tasty and filling meals while also benefiting from the many health advantages linked to fats derived from grass-fed animals, coconuts, and avocados.

Essentially, the Bulletproof Diet embraces a more complex view of dietary fats and challenges conventional wisdom by praising the function of high-quality fats as nutritional friends. The advantages impact not only physical health but also mental performance and stamina. One may improve their health and well-being in general by changing their diet to include a range of good fats from different sources.

High-Quality Proteins

An essential component of the Bulletproof Diet for reaching one's health and performance goals is the consumption of high-quality proteins. This dietary approach highlights the function of high-quality protein sources in boosting general well-being, acknowledging the importance of protein in numerous physiological processes.

Proteins are essential for many body processes, such as constructing muscles, supporting the immune system, and regulating hormones, among many others. In order to ensure that the body has access to the amino acids it needs to perform these tasks effectively, high-quality proteins become crucial. The Bulletproof method places an emphasis on the quality of the protein ingested rather than its amount, in contrast to conventional protein-centric diets.

In keeping with the principle of obtaining nutrient-dense, clean, and ethically farmed foods, the Bulletproof Diet suggests a wide range of protein sources. Prime examples of high-quality protein sources include beef and lamb that are grass-fed or reared on pasture. Not only do these cuts of beef supply the body with necessary amino acids, but they also have healthy fats like omega-3 and conjugated linoleic acid (CLA).

Protein-rich and rich in heart- and brain-healthy omega-3 fatty acids, wild-caught fish like mackerel and salmon are a great addition to any diet. Eggs that are reared on pasture are a great source of protein and other nutrients, including all nine essential amino acids and a host of vitamins and minerals.

With an eye on quality and bioavailability, the Bulletproof Diet also takes into account plant-based protein alternatives. For people who choose a plant-based diet, plant-based proteins such as quinoa, lentils, and beans can supplement their protein consumption.

Protein should come from clean, ethically farmed, and minimally processed sources; this is what the Bulletproof Diet stresses. People may help maintain a healthy metabolism and hormonal equilibrium while also aiding in muscle growth and recovery by making high-quality proteins a top priority.

Essentially, the Bulletproof Diet acknowledges that high-quality proteins are crucial for reaching one's health goals. It stresses the importance of both the amount and quality of protein sources, and it promotes a deliberate and contemplative approach to protein consumption. This diet allows participants to take advantage of all the nutritional powerhouses that proteins provide for optimal health and performance by including a wide variety of clean, ethically produced proteins.

Low-Toxin Vegetables

Incorporating low-toxin veggies is a key component of the Bulletproof Diet, which aims to improve health in general. By emphasizing the importance of selecting nutrient-dense vegetables while limiting exposure to possible contaminants, this dietary philosophy acknowledges that not all veggies are equal.

Crucial to the Bulletproof Diet are nutrient-dense veggies, which supply the body with antioxidants, vitamins, and minerals needed for a wide range of biological activities. The focus here is on the nutritional profile and quality of the veggies eaten, rather than just the amount. This method prioritizes nutrient-dense vegetables, such as dark greens like kale and spinach, cruciferous veggies like broccoli and cauliflower, and colorful alternatives like bell peppers.

Fundamental to the Bulletproof way of thinking is the idea of reducing dietary toxins. Pesticides and other chemicals used in conventional vegetable farming have the potential to upset the body's delicate equilibrium and cause systemic inflammation when consumed regularly. Individuals following the Bulletproof Diet strive to limit their intake of potentially dangerous chemicals by focusing on eating veggies that are organic and purchased locally. This allows their bodies to flourish on clean, healthy meals.

The Dirty Dozen and Clean Fifteen lists, which rank fruits and vegetables according to their pesticide residue levels, are essential to this strategy. The Bulletproof Diet recommends buying organic versions of the Dirty Dozen veggies to cut down on toxins even further. This well-planned strategy guarantees that people enjoy the health benefits of veggies while reducing their risk of exposure to harmful environmental pollutants.

In addition, there is a significance for cooking procedures in reducing toxins. To keep veggies' nutrients intact and reduce their exposure to potential surface contaminants, the Bulletproof Diet recommends steaming or sautéing them.

By emphasizing nutrient-dense alternatives and minimizing exposure to contaminants, the Bulletproof Diet essentially promotes a deliberate and thoughtful approach to eating vegetables. Individuals may enhance the health advantages of veggies while limiting dangers connected with environmental pollutants by selecting organic, locally produced food and being mindful of cooking procedures. Incorporating low-toxin veggies into the diet in this way supports the body's natural functions and optimizes overall health.

PART THREE: The Bulletproof Roadmap

If you want a detailed plan for improving your health and performance with food, go no further than the Bulletproof Diet. In order to feed the body efficiently, it stresses the consumption of high-quality fats, moderate proteins, and minimal carbs. Phase one of the plan involves replacing processed meals, sweets, and carbohydrates with Bulletproof Coffee and other nutrient-dense options. Diets are fine-tuned as people go along by responding to their unique needs and preferences by changing things like macronutrient ratios and when they eat. The diet promotes being present when eating by highlighting the importance of eating organic, complete foods and being aware of when you're full. Supplements are also encouraged as a means to improve health in general. The Bulletproof Diet is a plan that everyone can follow to get healthy and stay that way, thanks to its adaptable nature and focus on high-quality nourishment.

Roadmap Overview

Optimizing health and performance via nutrition is made easy with the comprehensive Bulletproof Diet road map. In order to feed the body efficiently, it emphasizes the consumption of high-quality fats, moderate proteins, and minimal carbohydrates. The first stage of the plan involves incorporating Bulletproof Coffee and nutrient-dense foods into your diet, while cutting out processed foods, sweets, and grains. As people go through life, they improve their eating habits by tailoring macronutrient ratios and meal timing to their own needs and preferences. The diet promotes mindful eating, with a focus on eating whole, organic foods and being mindful of hunger and satiety cues. In addition, it suggests taking vitamins to help with overall health. Optimal health and vitality may be achieved by following the Bulletproot Diet roadmap, which is known for its flexible approach and focus on quality nutrition.

Meal Planning in the Green Zone

The Bulletproof Diet's Green Zone is all about eating the right foods to keep you healthy, energized, and full of life. Incorporating nutrient-dense, anti-inflammatory foods into meal planning within this zone is all about reducing allergies and pollutants. Fats from grass-fed cows, coconuts, and avocados are the star of the show since they keep you going all day long and help your brain work better. Organic eggs, wild-caught salmon, and meats reared on pasture are good protein sources because they include the amino acids your muscles need to develop and repair. The high vitamin, mineral, and fiber content of non-starchy veggies, such as broccoli, cauliflower, and leafy greens, aids digestion and promotes good gut health. In order to maintain stable blood sugar levels and maintained energy throughout the day, meal planning entails making balanced, filling meals that mix these components in the right amounts. For even more metabolic flexibility and fat-burning potential, people may add Bulletproof Coffee or intermittent fasting to their diet programs. The Bulletproof Diet's Green Zone provides a road map to optimum nutrition and thriving health via meticulous consideration of food composition and component quality.

Managing Yellow Zone Foods

When it comes to meal selections in the Bulletproof Diet Yellow Zone, moderation and prudence are crucial. Allergy, sensitivity, and personal objectives are some of the variables that could affect how certain foods affect an individual's health and performance. Here you'll find grains, legumes, and fruits that some people may eat in moderation without experiencing negative side effects like inflammation or dangerously high blood sugar levels. To keep foods in the Yellow Zone under control, one must monitor their effects on vitality, disposition, and health in general. Identifying meals that are well-tolerated and those that should be limited or avoided may need experimentation and self-awareness. Controlling portions, eating them with fats and proteins to reduce their effect on blood sugar, and selecting the best sources are all ways to deal with foods that are in the Yellow Zone. Furthermore, it can be helpful for people to avoid acquiring sensitivities to foods in the Yellow Zone by rotating or cycling them. One way to stay on track and get the most out of the Bulletproof Diet is to be alert and careful while eating items that are in the Yellow Zone.

Understanding and Eliminating Red Zone Foods

For optimal health and performance, it's best to stay away from the items included in the Bulletproof Diet's Red Zone. Consumption of certain items, such as refined sugars, industrial seed oils, and artificial additives, can lead to hormone disruptions, impaired metabolic function, inflammation, and impaired gut health. To optimize health and achieve the desired outcomes from the diet, it is necessary to understand which foods are in the Red Zone and to eliminate them. Being attentive of the quality of materials used in cooking and meal preparation, reading labels carefully to uncover hidden substances, and if feasible, choosing whole, unprocessed alternatives are all part of this. The meals that fall into the "Red Zone" category tend to be heavy in calories without nutrients and can have negative effects on digestive health and immunity. People can improve their health in general, lower inflammation, and regulate blood sugar levels by cutting out certain items from their diet. Meal prepping, cooking in bulk, and having Bulletproof-approved substitutes for frequent offenders like processed grains, hydrogenated oils, and artificial sweeteners are all great ways to cut out Red Zone items from your diet. By being committed and mindful, anybody may successfully complete the Bulletproof Diet's Red Zone, leading to enhanced health and vigor.

Sample Meal Plans

To help you put the Bulletproof Diet's concepts into practice in your daily life, the diet includes sample meal plans. Goals of these programs include maximizing energy and performance, promoting fullness, and stabilizing blood sugar levels. Bulletproof Coffee, prepared with premium coffee beans, grass-fed butter, and MCT oil or coconut oil, is a common morning beverage on the

Bulletproof Diet. It provides energy and improves focus. An example of a protein-and fat-rich breakfast might be grass-fed butter fried pasture-raised eggs with sliced avocado and sautéed spinach. A big salad of mixed greens, grilled chicken or fish gathered in the wild, with a dressing of olive oil and apple cider vinegar may be lunch. A handful of raw nuts (almonds, macadamia nuts, etc.) with some berries or grass-fed cheese would make a great mid-day snack. Dinner may be a well-rounded affair with grass-fed beef or bison burgers encased in lettuce leaves, accompanied by roasted veggies mixed with coconut oil and herbs. A modest portion of mixed berries topped with whipped coconut cream or a piece of dark chocolate with a high cocoa content are dessert alternatives on the Bulletproof Diet. People may experience the health advantages of the Bulletproof Diet and savor tasty, filling meals

by following these sample meal plans.

PART FOUR: DELICIOUS BULLETPROOF DIET RECIPES

DELICIOUS BULLETPROOF DIET BREAKSAT RECIPS

FLUFFY ALMOND FLOUR AND VANILLA PANCAKES

INGREDIENTS

1 cup blanched almond flour

2 eggs

2-3 tbsp sweetener of your choice

3 tbsp melted butter or ghee or avocado oil

1 scoop collagen protein powder

2 tsp vanilla extract

1/4 tsp. baking soda

1/2 tsp. apple cider vinegar or lemon juice

Chocolate Sauce

1/4 – 1/3 block high-quality dark chocolate, 78% cacao or higher

3/4 tbsp. butter or ghee or avocado oil

3/4 tbsp. coconut oil

1/2 tbsp. sweetener of your choice

Optional Toppings

Berries

A drizzle of honey or pure maple syrup

INSTRUCTIONS

Preheat a pan over medium-low heat on the stove. As it heats, stir together all of the ingredients, keeping in mind that the batter won't be quite as runny as traditional pancake batter. When the batter is too wet, the pancakes are difficult to flip, so don't add any extra water to thin out the mixture.

Grease the preheated pan with butter, Grass-Fed Ghee or oil, then pour 1/4 cup of the batter into the center of the pan. Shake the pan gently to encourage the batter to spread out a little.

Cook until little bubbles start to form, and as soon as the bottom feels sturdy enough to flip (about 3 to 4 minutes of cooking time), use a spatula to flip the pancake and cook the other side until golden brown.

Repeat with the remaining batter, until all of the pancakes are cooked. You should get four medium sized pancakes or seven to eight smaller pancakes.

Now add all of the chocolate sauce ingredients into a small saucepan. Melt on low-medium heat and stir together until fully melted.

Place the pancakes onto two plates, top with berries and drizzle the chocolate sauce over the top, or serve warm with your favorite toppings.

SMOKED SALMON AND GARLIC SPINACH

INGREDIENTS

4 tbsp. coconut oil

8 slices of your preferred sandwich vessel (like Cauliflower Sandwich Thins)

4 oz. smoked salmon

9 oz. fresh spinach

4 tbsp. organic powdered eggs, or 2 whole pasture-raised eggs

4 tbsp. water

2 cloves garlic or 1/2 tsp. garlic powder

1/2 lemon

INSTRUCTIONS

If using powdered eggs, hydrate them in water. Stir and let sit for 5 minutes.

Meanwhile, turn on burner to medium heat. Add 2 tbsp. coconut oil to pan.

Toast sandwich bread on both sides. While the bread is toasting, mince the garlic cloves.

Once all slices have been toasted, add remaining 2 tbsp. of coconut oil to pan. Cook garlic 1-2 minutes. Add spinach, and cook 2-3 minutes until wilted.

Add eggs. Stir, scrambling gently and cooking 2-3 minutes until set. Finish with a squeeze of lemon.

Layer smoked salmon and garlic spinach scramble on toast. Eat!

KETO COFFEE CAKE

INGREDIENTS

KETO COFFEE CAKE

2 cups almond flour

1 cup coconut flour

3 eggs

1/2 cup coconut milk

1/2 cup Bulletproof Grass-Fed Ghee (melted)

1/4 cup quality birchwood xylitol or erythritol

2 tsp lemon juice or apple cider vinegar

2 tsp vanilla extract

1 tsp cinnamon

1 tsp baking soda

STREUSEL TOPPING

 1/2 tsp cinnamon

1-1 1/2 tbsp quality birchwood xylitol or erythritol

1 tbsp coconut flour

2-3 tbsp Bulletproof Grass-Fed Ghee (softened)

5-6 tbsp almond flour

GLAZE (OPTIONAL)

1 tbsp Bulletproof Vanilla Collagen Protein

1-3 tsp powdered birchwood xylitol or erythritol

1 tbsp Bulletproof Brain Octane C8 MCT Oil

2 tbsp almond butter

1/2 tsp vanilla extract

INSTRUCTIONS

Preheat the oven to 340°F (170°C). Grease and line a cake pan with parchment paper.

Add all the cake **Ingredients** into a bowl or food processor and combine evenly.

Scoop the mixture into the prepared cake tin and spread out evenly. Note the mixture will be quite thick, due to the coconut flour.

Add all the streusel **Ingredients** into the same bowl or food processor and mix or blend until crumbs form. If the mixture is too wet, add in 1 Tbsp. more of almond flour and pulse together until a 'crumb' texture is achieved.

Evenly sprinkle the streusel mixture on top of the cake.

Place into the oven and bake for 45 minutes or until the cake is thoroughly baked. When it looks ready, turn the oven off, leave the cake inside the oven but leave the door ajar.

Add all of the glaze **Ingredients**into a small bowl and whisk together.

Once the cake has cooled, drizzle some of the glaze over the top and serve with a piping-hot cup of clean Bulletproof Coffee.

PASTURE-RAISED EGG BITES

INGREDIENTS

7 oz chemical-free, free-range bacon (diced)

2 bunches scallions (chopped)

1 rosemary sprig (finely chopped)

 1/2 zucchini squash (finely diced)

8 pasture-raised eggs

1 tbsp Bulletproof Grass-Fed Ghee

2 scoops Bulletproof Unflavored Collagen Protein

1 tsp Himalayan pink salt

INSTRUCTIONS

Preheat oven to 350F°. Line standard muffin tin with parchment paper, or use silicone muffin tray.

Heat frying pan over medium heat. Add bacon and rosemary, and fry until golden-brown. Add zucchini and continue cooking for a few more minutes, then turn off heat. Stir chopped scallions through.

Add eggs, collagen protein, salt and ghee into a blender.

Pour egg mixture into muffin tray cavities. Spoon bacon and veggie mixture on top, evenly.

Place muffin tray in oven, and bake for 25-30 minutes, or until fully cooked.

Remove from oven and enjoy warm.

Optional: Once cooled, store in freezer-safe container. Reheat, as needed.

COLLAGEN BREAKFAST COOKIES

INGREDIENTS

2 eggs

1/2 cup almond flour

1/2 cup shredded coconut

1/2 cup sliced almonds

1/2 cup pecans

1/2 cup pumpkin seeds

1/2 cup sugar-free chocolate chips

1/3 cup roasted almond butter

1/3 cup granulated monk fruit-erythritol blend

2 tbsp ground flax meal

2 1/2 tbsp Bulletproof Vanilla Collagen Protein

2-3 tsp cinnamon

2-3 tsp ginger powder

1 tsp vanilla extract

INSTRUCTIONS

Preheat oven to 350°F.

Line two baking trays with parchment paper.

Mix all cookie ingredients together in a bowl.

Oil hands with some coconut oil and roll the mixture into balls. Place them on the lined baking trays and press them into flat, even cookies.

Place the tray in the oven and bake for approximately 20-25 minutes, or until golden and cooked through.

Remove cookies from oven and allow time to cool.

Serve with a hot cup of Bulletproof Coffee for a keto-friendly breakfast!

KETO ICED COFFEE PROTEIN SHAKE

INGREDIENTS

1/2 avocado (or 1/4 large avocado) frozen with skin and pit removed

4 oz Bulletproof Original Coffee brewed and frozen into cubes

1 1/4 cup unsweetened full-fat coconut milk (or milk of choice)

1 scoop Bulletproof Vanilla Collagen Peptides

1/2 tbsp Bulletproof Brain Octane C8 MCT Oil

1 tbsp cacao powder

1/4 tsp Ceylon cinnamon

1/2 cup ice (in addition to cold brew cubes)

INSTRUCTIONS

Add all ingredients to a blender. Blend, starting on
a low speed and working your way up.

Garnish, if desired, and serve.

KETO PANCAKE CEREAL

INGREDIENTS

1 cup blanched almond flour

2 eggs

2-3 Tbsp. sweetener of your choice

3 Tbsp. melted butter or ghee or avocado oil

1 scoop Collagen Protein powder

2 tsp. vanilla extract

1/4 tsp. baking soda

1/2 tsp. apple cider vinegar or lemon juice

INSTRUCTIONS

Combine all of the pancake ingredients. The batter won't be as runny as traditional pancake batter, but resist the urge to add more liquid.

Heat a pan over medium heat until uniformly hot. Grease the pan coconut oil, butter or Grass-Fed Ghee.

Add batter to a battery bottle or bag with the corner cut for easier dispensing.

Arrange nickel-sized pancakes around the bottom of the pan, being careful not to crowd the pan. You'll need space to flip the little guys.

Flip each pancake after about 3 to 4 minutes. Cook on the second side for about 2 more minutes or until cooked through.

Add cooked pancakes to a bowl and top with butter. They would also be delicious with almond butter, almond milk or fruit compote.

GRAIN-FREE GRANOLA

INGREDIENTS

1 1/2 cups pumpkin seeds

1 cup sunflower seeds

2 cups almonds, roughly chopped

1 cup cashews, roughly chopped

1 cup Brazil nuts, roughly chopped

1 cup pistachios

3-4 Tbsp. melted coconut oil

3-5 Tbsp. honey (or sugar-free sweetener of your choice)

2-3 tsp. Ceylon cinnamon powder

1 cup shredded coconut

1 cup coconut flakes

2 Bulletproof Collagen Protein Bars, diced and mixed through the final granola (optional)

INSTRUCTIONS

Preheat your oven to 340°F / 170°C.

Add everything into a bowl (except the dried coconut and optional Collagen Protein Bars). Mix together evenly.

Spread the nuts out onto a baking tray evenly. Place into the oven and bake for 15 minutes.

Remove from the oven and mix the nuts and seeds together and spread it out evenly again. Place it back into the oven and bake for another 15 minutes.

Remove from the oven and stir the dried coconut through the nut and seed mix evenly. Place it back into the oven and bake for 5 minutes. Remove from the oven. If the nuts, seeds and coconut are all toasted evenly, you can remove from the oven and allow to cool completely. Or if it needs another 5 minutes to toast that little bit more, place it back into the oven to finish off.

Remove from oven once the granola is toasted to your preference. If you're adding in the chopped Bulletproof Collagen Bars, mix them through. Store in a glass jar once completely cool.

Serve with coconut yogurt and seasonal fruit or berries, enjoy as a snack, mix it through cookie dough or muffin mix and bake or sprinkle over homemade gluten-free pancakes or Bulletproof ice cream for a crunchy topping.

SMOKED SALMON AND GARLIC SPINACH BREAKFAST SANDWICH

INGREDIENTS

4 tbsp. coconut oil

8 slices of your preferred sandwich vessel (like Cauliflower Sandwich Thins)

4 oz. smoked salmon

9 oz. fresh spinach

4 tbsp. organic powdered eggs, or 2 whole pasture-raised eggs

4 tbsp. water

2 cloves garlic or 1/2 tsp. garlic powder

1/2 lemon

INSTRUCTIONS

If using powdered eggs, hydrate them in water. Stir and let sit for 5 minutes.

Meanwhile, turn on burner to medium heat. Add 2 tbsp. coconut oil to pan.

Toast sandwich bread on both sides. While the bread is toasting, mince the garlic cloves.

Once all slices have been toasted, add remaining 2 tbsp. of coconut oil to pan. Cook garlic 1-2 minutes. Add spinach, and cook 2-3 minutes until wilted.

Add eggs. Stir, scrambling gently and cooking 2-3 minutes until set. Finish with a squeeze of lemon.

Layer smoked salmon and garlic spinach scramble on toast. Eat!

KETO COCONUT FLOUR PANCAKES

INGREDIENTS

1/2 cup (50g) coconut flour

1/2 tsp baking soda

2 tbsp coconut oil, melted

4 organic, pasture raised eggs, room temperature

1 tsp vanilla

1/2 tsp Ceylon cinnamon

1/2 cup coconut cream (the thick part of canned coconut cream, unsweetened)

1/2 cup almond milk, unsweetened

1/4 tsp Himalayan salt

Grass-fed Ghee or coconut oil for cooking

INSTRUCTIONS

In a high-powered blender, add all **Ingredient** sexcept ghee and blend until well incorporated, scraping the sides down as needed.

Heat a medium skillet over medium heat, then add enough ghee to coat the pan. When pan has heated, pour about 1/2 cup of batter onto the skillet. Cook batter until golden on one side, then flip and continue cooking until golden on the other side (note: Thicker pancakes will take longer to cook). Set aside and continue cooking until no batter remains.

Serve coconut flour pancakes hot with grass-fed ghee, berries, or your favorite keto-friendly toppings.

DELICIOUS BULLET PROOF DIET MAIN DISH RECIPS

PUMPKIN SPICE KETO GRANOLA RECIPE

INGREDIENTS

1 cup sunflower seeds

1 cup pumpkin seeds

1 cup pecans

1 cup almonds (chopped)

1 cup cashews (chopped)

1/2 cup Brazil nuts (chopped)

2 cups coconut flakes (unsweetened)

3 tbsp granulated sweetener, such as non-GMO erythritol or birch xylitol

3 tbsp Bulletproof Grass-Fed Ghee

2 tbsp Bulletproof Brain Octane C8 MCT Oil

1 scoop Bulletproof Unflavored Collagen Protein

1-2 tsp vanilla extract

1 tbsp pumpkin pie spice

INSTRUCTIONS

Preheat oven to 320ºF. Line a large baking tray with parchment paper.

Add all **Ingredients** into a large bowl (except for the collagen powder) and mix until everything is evenly coated.

Pour onto the lined baking sheet evenly, place into the oven and bake for 15 minutes.

Remove tray from oven, toss the mixture so all sides get evenly toasted and place back into oven to bake for another 7-10 minutes, or until golden brown. NOTE: Be sure to keep an eye on it so your keto granola recipe doesn't burn!

Remove from oven and stir in the collagen protein powder while the granola is still warm.

Allow to cool completely before transferring to a large glass jar or airtight container to store at room temperature.

For a quick keto breakfast, serve in a bowl with your milk of choice, atop a heap of probiotic coconut yogurt and berries, or for added crunch to your morning smoothie bowl.

GREEN SHAKSHUKA RECIPE

INGREDIENTS

3-4 tbsp Bulletproof Grass-Fed Ghee

4 garlic cloves (finely chopped)

1 zucchini (diced)

1 tsp cumin

1/2 tsp salt

1 bunch kale (de-stemmed and chopped)

5-6 large eggs

 1/4 cup fresh cilantro or parsley (chopped)

1 avocado (large, sliced for garnish)

INSTRUCTIONS

Heat 1-2 tbsp ghee in a frying pan on medium heat.

Add the diced zucchini and cook until it has some color.

Add 2 tbsp ghee into the pan to melt along with the garlic, chopped greens and salt. Cover with lid and allow everything to steam for a few minutes.

Give the mix a good stir. When the greens have softened, flatten the mixture with a spatula and create 5-6 small wells.

Crack the eggs into each well and cook until they are done to your liking. (Hint: Use the lid to create steam and speed up the process!)

Sprinkle fresh herbs on top, garnish with sliced avocado and add extra salt, if desired.

Serve up a portion of this green shakshuka recipe, dig in and enjoy!

CREAMY AVOCADO PESTO

INGREDIENTS

2 avocados

1 cup fresh basil (or use a mixture of basil and coriander)

Juice from 1/2 a lemon

1 garlic clove (optional)

2-3 Tbsp Bulletproof Brain Octane oil

2-3 Tbsp water

Salt to taste

INSTRUCTIONS

Combine all **Ingredients**together in a food processor until combined. Scrape down the sides of the bowl and re-blend.

Mix the pesto through zoodles, spread on homemade gluten-free toast, serve with roast chicken or use as a dip with roasted sweet potato fries.

Avocado Dressing (Creamy and Vegan)

INGREDIENTS

1 avocado

2 tsp lime juice freshly squeezed

1/2 tsp salt

1/2 cup almond milk (adjust for texture preference)

2 Tbsp water

1 tsp black pepper (optional)

INSTRUCTIONS

In a food processor, add 1 avocado that is peeled and roughly chopped

Add 2 tsp of freshly squeezed lime juice

Add 1 tsp of salt and black pepper. Black pepper is optional

Add 1/2 cup of almond milk. If you prefer creamier, add more almond milk

Add 2 Tbsp of water and blend on low speed until it is well blended

Transfer to a bottle and refrigerate for 30 minutes. You can store it for up to 2 weeks in the fridge

Other **Ingredients** you can add to this dressing: Red onions, roasted garlic, tarragon, olive oil, cilantro or dill.

Bacon-Wrapped Avocado Fries

Ingredients

2 avocados

20 strips of pasture-raised bacon

Instructions

Preheat the oven to 425ºF and line a baking sheet with parchment paper. Remove the pits from the avocados and slice the avocado into thin strips lengthwise (5 per half).

Wrap each avocado slice with one strip of bacon, and place on the baking sheet. Bake for 25-30 minutes or until the bacon is crisp. Allow to cool for 5 minutes before serving.

NO-BEAN KETO CHILI

INGREDIENTS

1 lb grass-fed ground beef (or lamb)

4 garlic cloves (minced)

1 onion (finely diced)

1 cup chicken or beef broth

1 zucchini (finely diced)

2 tbsp tomato paste

2 tsp chili powder

1 tsp cayenne pepper

1 tsp cumin

1 tsp salt

1/2 tsp black pepper

1/2 tsp chili flakes

1-2 tbsp Bulletproof Collagelatin

2 tbsp Bulletproof Grass-Fed Ghee

1 cup coconut yogurt (garnish)

1 tsp fresh herbs (garnish)

INSTRUCTIONS

Heat frying pan over medium heat. Add 1 tablespoon of Grass-Fed Ghee and fry the diced onion and minced garlic until golden-brown.

Add another tablespoon of Ghee and ground beef (or lamb) and sauté until meat is browned.

Add spices, zucchini, salt, pepper, tomato paste and broth. Stir to combine, and simmer for 30 minutes to 1 hour. Speed up the thickening process by adding 1-2 tablespoons of Collagelatin.

Taste the mixture and add additional chili powder or cayenne pepper, if desired.

Ladle into a bowl, garnish with chives and chili flakes, top with coconut yogurt and enjoy!

PALEO CAULIFLOWER FRITTERS

INGREDIENTS

1 large cauliflower head, broken into florets

1/3 cup Collagen Peptides

1/3 cup coconut flour

2 pasture-raised eggs

1 teaspoon baking soda

1/2 teaspoon ground turmeric

1/2 teaspoon ground ginger

1/2 teaspoon ground cinnamon

1 tablespoon Grass-Fed Ghee

Fresh cilantro to garnish

Salt to taste

INSTRUCTIONS

In a steamer basket with 1 inch of boiling water, steam cauliflower florets until tender. Then, allow to cool on a plate while preparing the other ingredients.

In a blender, add cauliflower and pulse until it forms a rice-like texture. Pour into a clean kitchen towel and gently squeeze out some of the excess water.

Transfer cauliflower to a mixing bowl and then add remaining **Ingredients** except cilantro. Mix well until combined.

In a skillet on medium heat, add ghee and allow it to melt around the pan.

Using your hands, shape cauliflower mixture into 6 fritters. Add fritters to pan and cook for 4-5 minutes. Carefully flip and cook for an additional 4-5 minutes.

Serve cauliflower fritters warm with salt and cilantro to taste.

KETO EGGS BENEDICT

INGREDIENTS

1/4 cup coconut flour

4 eggs, beaten

1/4 cup full-fat canned coconut milk (BPA-free)

1/2 teaspoon baking soda

1/2 teaspoon salt

HOLLANDAISE SAUCE **INGREDIENTS**

3 egg yolks

1 1/2 tablespoons water

1/2 cup plus 2 tablespoons cold grass-fed butter, cut into small pieces

Salt to taste

2 teaspoons lemon juice

POACHED EGG **INGREDIENTS**

6 ounces wild-caught smoked salmon

8 pastured eggs

1 tablespoon apple cider vinegar or lemon juice

Thinly sliced chives to garnish

INSTRUCTIONS

Prepare English muffins first. In a small bowl, whisk together all muffin **Ingredients**until smooth.

Divide batter evenly into four medium heat-safe ramekins. Bake at 350 degrees for 5-10 minutes, or until a toothpick inserted comes out clean.

Prepare hollandaise sauce. Fill a medium saucepan with one inch of water. Bring water up to a simmer over medium high heat, then reduce to a gentle simmer.

Add egg yolks and water to a medium glass bowl that can sit on top of the saucepan without falling in or touching the water. Set the bowl over the pan and whisk the egg mixture constantly until it lightens and thickens (about 1-2 minutes).

Gradually mix in pieces of butter, allow them to melt one by one.

Remove hollandaise from heat and whisk until completely smooth, placing it back on the simmering saucepan as needed to keep warm. Season with salt and lemon juice. When warmed, pour sauce in a thermos to retain temperature.

Prepare poached eggs. Bring a saucepan filled with water to a boil. Reduce the heat to bring it to a gentle simmer. Add vinegar.

In a pinch bowl, crack one egg.

Using a spoon, stir water in a clockwise circle to create a whirlpool in the center of the pot.

When whirlpool has formed, carefully pour the egg into the center of the whirlpool so egg whites wrap around the yolk as it spins. Cook for 5 minutes. (If you're already familiar with poaching eggs and have a large enough pan, you can cook up to four at once.)

Using a slotted spoon, remove eggs from pot and place on a paper towel to drain. Repeat as needed until all eggs are poached.

Assemble keto eggs Benedict. Slice and lightly toast English muffins, then add two muffin pieces to each plate. Top each slice with slices of smoked salmon, one poached egg, hollandaise sauce, and a sprinkle of chives. Serve immediately.

PALEO SWEET POTATO NACHOS

INGREDIENTS

2 sweet potatoes, thinly sliced

600 grams ground lamb

2 spring onions, sliced

1 onion, diced

4 garlic cloves, crushed

1 tomato, finely chopped

1-2 Tbsp. tomato paste (no added salt)

1 Tbsp. bone broth powder (optional)

Handful of coriander leaves or parsley, chopped

1/2 - 1 Tbsp. taco seasoning

2 ripe avocados, diced

Lemon or lime juice, to taste

1/2 Tbsp. quality olive oil

Salt to taste

Coconut oil for shallow frying

Tip: For next-level guacamole, use Brain Octane MCT oil instead of olive oil.

INSTRUCTIONS

Preheat a frying pan with some coconut oil. Add the onion and sauté until golden brown. Then add the ground lamb and begin to brown.

Add the tomato paste, chopped tomato, spring onion, taco seasoning, bone broth powder (if using), coriander or parsley and garlic and stir through. Allow this to simmer and thicken while you begin shallow frying the sweet potato chips.

Heat a large frying pan with some coconut oil. Working in batches, begin to shallow fry the sweet potato slices until golden brown and crispy. Carefully remove them from the pan once they're ready. Place them onto a lined tray to drip-dry. Continue cooking all of the sweet potato chips.

Check the ground lamb. Give it a stir to prevent the bottom from sticking to the pan.

In a small bowl, add the chopped avocado, lemon or lime juice, salt to taste and a drizzle of quality olive oil (or MCT oil) and stir to combine.

Once the chips are all cooked and the mince is nice and thick, remove it from the heat and begin plating. Garnish with some fresh coriander or parsley. Serve and enjoy.

EASY SLOW-COOKED LAMB BARBACOA

INGREDIENTS

5 lamb shanks or 2 pounds lamb shoulder (room temperature)

1 cup bone broth

1 tbsp. smoked paprika

1 tbsp. ground cumin

1 tbsp. dried oregano

2 tsp. garlic powder or 4-5 cloves of garlic, finely chopped

1 1/2 - 2 tsp. chipotle powder

1 tsp. salt

1/2 tsp. ceylon cinnamon powder

A drizzle of Brain Octane C8 MCT Oil

INSTRUCTIONS

In a small mixing bowl, add all the spices and salt. Stir to combine.

Add the lamb roast or shanks into your slow cooker or, if you're cooking in the oven, place it in an ovenproof dish. Evenly distribute the spice mix over the lamb. Make sure to get it into all of the crevices as best you can.

Slow cooker: Pour the bone broth into the slow cooker and turn the heat to high. Cook for 5-6 hours. Oven: If you're using the oven, pour the bone broth into the ovenproof dish and place into a preheated oven. Cook for 6 hours at 110°C or 230°F.

When fully cooked, the lamb should shred easily with two forks. Shred the lamb and remove the bones (save them to make homemade bone broth).

Optional, to serve as carnitas: Turn the oven up to 180°C or 350°F. If you've cooked the lamb in your slow cooker, add it to an ovenproof dish. Add the lamb into the oven to cook for a further 10-15 minutes, or until some of the lamb on top begins to go crispy.

When it's ready, serve the meat wrapped in lettuce, homemade tortillas or wraps with your favorite toppings. After plating, finish with a drizzle of Brain Octane C8 MCT Oil (optional, but recommended).

SLOW-BAKED SALMON AND VEGGIE BOWL

INGREDIENTS

2 cups spinach

14 green beans, trimmed

1/2 sweet potato, sliced into chips

6-8 broccoli florets

1/2 large avocado, sliced

15 oz. boneless wild-caught salmon (room temperature)

Optional: 1 tbsp. wild-caught salmon roe (with no colors or preservatives)

1-2 tbsp. Grass-Fed Ghee or butter, melted

A drizzle of cold-pressed olive oil or Brain Octane MCT oil

Lemon wedges to serve

Salt to taste

INSTRUCTIONS

Preheat the oven to 355°F. Line a baking tray with parchment paper.

Add the sweet potato chips onto the lined baking tray. Add 1/2 to 1 tbsp. melted butter or ghee and a little sprinkle of salt. Mix so they're coated evenly. Place into the oven and bake for 10 minutes.

Meanwhile, set a steamer basket in a small-medium saucepan filled with 2 inches of water. Add the green beans and steam for roughly four to five minutes. Add in the broccoli florets and cook for another four to five minutes. (The time will depend on how tender or crisp you like them, so please keep an eye on them.) Remove from the heat when they're cooked.

Check the sweet potato chips and turn them over using some tongs. Continue cooking for a few more minutes. Once the sweet potato chips are ready, remove them from the oven.

Turn the oven down to 275°F.

Pat salmon dry with a paper towel and place onto a lined baking tray. Use a pastry brush to brush the salmon with the melted butter or ghee. You can also add your favorite seasonings or marinade here if desired. Sprinkle a little salt on top. Place into the oven and cook for 15-20 minutes (the time will depend on how big the salmon is). You can test with a fork in the middle of the fish. If it flakes easily, it's ready.

Remove the salmon from the oven. You can pop the veggies into the oven for a few minutes to reheat while you begin plating.

Place the spinach leaves onto two plates. Add the sliced avocado on top, followed by the salmon and veggies. Drizzle with cold pressed olive oil or

Brain Octane MCT oil and lemon juice. Add the optional salmon roe on top. Enjoy!

DELICIOUS BULLETPROOF DIET DESSERT RECIPES

HAZELNUT KETO FUDGESICLES

INGREDIENTS

1 cup coconut yogurt

1 avocado

1 tbsp Bulletproof Chocolate Collagen Peptides

1 tbsp Bulletproof Hazelnut Creamer

2 tbsp Bulletproof Brain Octane C8 MCT Oil (can also use Bulletproof MCT Oil)

3-4 tbsp cacao powder

1 tsp vanilla extract

2-4 tbsp granulated monk fruit

 1/2 cup cashews

1 tsp cinnamon

INSTRUCTIONS

Add all **Ingredients** into a blender and blitz until completely smooth.

Scrape down the sides and blend again to make sure there are no lumps. Taste the mixture and add more sweetener, if needed.

Pour into the molds (we made five popsicles) and insert the pop sticks.

Place in the freezer for 4-5 hours, or overnight.

Once frozen, remove from the freezer, pop out of the molds and decorate with melted chocolate, a sprinkle of homemade granola or fresh berries, based on your flavor preferences.

KETO TRES LECHES CAKE

INGREDIENTS

CAKE

2 1/2 cups blanched almond flour

¾ cup unsalted butter (or Bulletproof Grass-Fed Ghee)

1/2 cup coconut flour

1/2 cup coconut milk

1/2 cup monk fruit (brown)

6 eggs

1 tsp vanilla powder (or 1 tbsp vanilla extract)

2 tsp baking soda

1 tbsp lemon juice

TRES LECHES (HOMEMADE CONDENSED COCONUT MILK)

27 oz coconut cream (available in 13.5 oz cans)

2-3 tbsp monk fruit (brown)

1 scoop Bulletproof Vanilla Bean Energy Collagen Protein

1 tsp vanilla extract

COCONUT WHIPPED CREAM

27 oz coconut cream (Put cans in refrigerator to cause cream to solidify and separate from the milk)

1-2 tbsp monk fruit (brown)

1 scoop Bulletproof French Vanilla Creamer

INSTRUCTIONS

Preheat oven to 350ºF.

Mix all the cake **Ingredients** together in a large bowl using a hand mixer.

Pour into an 8x8 greased, parchment-lined dish or a rectangle/slice tin.

Bake for 30 minutes or until cooked through and golden.

Meanwhile, make the tres leches by adding condensed milk, vanilla and sweetener into a medium-sized saucepan and bring the mix to a soft boil. Reduce for 30 minutes or until it's reduced by half and has thickened. Stir occasionally, especially toward the end to prevent the mixture from burning on the bottom.

Once the cake is finished baking, allow it cool.

Once the homemade condensed coconut milk is ready and off the heat, add Vanilla Bean Energy Collagen Protein and whisk until combined.

Poke the top of the cake to make a lot of holes and pour the condensed coconut milk mixture over the top so the cake absorbs all that tasty goodness.

Place cake in the refrigerator to set. Place a heavy mixing bowl (or the bowl from your stand mixer) in the freezer to chill for the coconut whipped cream.

Add the solid coconut cream to the chilled mixing bowl and use a hand mixer or stand mixer to whip it. Add sweetener of choice and French Vanilla Creamer and continue whipping until the cream stiffens.

Spread the coconut whipped cream evenly over the cake and top with fresh berries. Once you dig into a slice of this keto tres leches cake recipe, you may never go back to the traditional version.

KETO BACON CHOCOLATE CHIP COOKIES

INGREDIENTS

2 cups almond flour finely ground

3 Tbsp. Bulletproof Grass-Fed Ghee or grass-fed butter

3 Tbsp. Bulletproof Unflavored Collagen Peptides

2 Tbsp. granulated non-GMO erythritol or birch xylitol (add more, if desired)

2 tsp. vanilla

1 egg

1/2 tsp. paleo-friendly baking powder

1 tsp. apple cider vinegar

1 pinch of salt

1/3 cup chocolate chips or chunks with at least 85% cacao

4 slices cooked and cooled pastured bacon, diced finely or crumbled

INSTRUCTIONS

Preheat oven to 340ºF.

Line two baking trays with parchment paper.

In a mixing bowl, add almond flour, collagen, sweetener and salt. Mix together, then add baking powder to the top.

Pour apple cider vinegar on top of the baking powder so it reacts (you'll see it bubble and fizz).

Add ghee, vanilla and egg and mix thoroughly. Add chocolate and bacon pieces, and mix once more.

Roll the dough into balls and place on the lined baking trays.

Press the balls flat into cookie shapes. Press flatter for a crunchier cookie, and leave more rounded for a softer, chewier cookie.

Bake for 15 minutes, or until golden.

Remove trays from oven and gently place cookies on a wire rack to cool.

When cooled, store leftover bacon chocolate chip
cookies in a covered container.

KETO COCONUT MACAROONS

INGREDIENTS

1 1/2 cup shredded coconut unsweetened

5 tbsp birch xylitol

1 scoop Bulletproof Vanilla Collagen Protein

1/2 tsp baking powder (aluminum-free)

1/2 tsp pure almond extract

2 egg whites patured

unsweetened dark chocolate baking chips Optional

INSTRUCTIONS

Preheat oven to 325ºF.

Place all of the dry **Ingredients** in a mixing bowl and stir well to evenly mix.

Add almond extract and egg whites and stir well to combine.

Use a large spoon to scoop nine equal servings and place them evenly spread apart on a parchment-lined (or silicone baking mat lined) baking sheet. If unlined, you will need to brush your baking sheet with oil to keep the macaroons from sticking.

Optional: Top each macaroon with a few unsweetened dark chocolate chips before placing in the oven.

Bake for approximately 15 minutes or until macaroons are lightly browned.

Using a spatula, remove from baking sheet and allow to cool before eating.

KETO S'MORES

INGREDIENTS

KETO MARSHMALLOWS

4 Tbsp. Bulletproof Collagelatin

1 cup water

2 Tbsp. birch xylitol

1/4 - 1/2 tsp. vanilla powder

KETO GRAHAM CRACKER COCONUT SHORTBREAD

3/4 cup + 1 Tbsp. coconut flour

3/4 cup Bulletproof Grass-Fed Ghee or butter, diced and cold

1/2 tsp. baking soda

2-3 Tbsp. birch xylitol

KETO CHOCOLATE

2 squares of your keto-friendly chocolate bar of choice

INSTRUCTIONS

MARSHMALLOWS

Add the Collagelatin and water into a saucepan. Whisk to combine and remove any lumps. Set aside for a few minutes to allow the Collagelatin to absorb some of the water.

Add the xylitol and vanilla into the saucepan on low-medium heat for a few minutes, or until the Collagelatin and xylitol has completely dissolved.

Remove from the heat, and allow to cool for 2-3 minutes.

Using an electric beater,, beat the mixture for approximately 8 minutes, or until the marshmallow mixture has increased in size and looks silky smooth, glossy and has some small bubbles. Tip: If the mixture cools down too quickly and you beat the mix for too long, it may begin to set and form a slightly chunky texture. Don't worry, though. Simply pop the saucepan back onto the stovetop and heat for 30 seconds-1 minute on very-low heat to melt a bit. Then, stir together. Remove from heat and beat again for a few more minutes, until the marshmallow mix is silky-smooth, glossy and has small bubbles forming.

Pour the mixture into a lined bread loaf tin, or a container of a similar size.

Place in the fridge to set, approximately 1 hour.

KETO GRAHAM CRACKER COCONUT SHORTBREAD

Preheat the oven to 350°F. Line a baking tray with parchment paper.

Add coconut flour, ghee (or cold, cubed butter), xylitol and baking soda into a food processor, and blitz to combine evenly. Blend in 1/2-1 Tbsp. of extra coconut flour, if needed; try not to add more, as the coconut flour will absorb the butter (liquid) after a few minutes.

Place a piece of parchment paper on the countertop. Use a spatula to get the dough out of the food processor and place it on top of the parchment paper. Shape it into a 'rough' rectangle. Place another piece of parchment paper on top, and use a rolling pin to roll it out into an even rectangle.

Use a knife to slice the dough into 12 squares or rectangles (approximately the size of 4 or 6 squares of a standard chocolate bar) and remove the excess, uneven edges of the dough. Re-roll the excess dough.

Place the tray of pre-sliced coconut shortbread graham squares into the oven, and bake for 12-13 minutes, or until golden-brown.

Once the shortbread is cooked, remove it from the oven and allow it to cool completely. DO NOT TOUCH until it has cooled completely, or it will crumble.

ASSEMBLY

Remove the marshmallow mixture from the fridge and bring to room temperature (these marshmallows have the best texture when at room temperature).

Preheat the oven to 250°F.

Once the graham cracker shortbread has cooled and set, place three of the squares onto a lined baking tray. Place 4-6 squares (whichever fits best on top) of your keto-friendly chocolate bar on top of the shortbread. Pop it into the oven for 1-2 minutes, or until you can visibly see the chocolate beginning to melt. Please keep an eye on it, as the chocolate may melt quickly.

Remove from the oven.

Remove the marshmallow slab from the tin or container. Place one of the shortbread squares or rectangles on top and cut around so you have the perfect-size marshmallow for the shortbread. Continue with the rest of the assembly.

Once all the components are ready, sandwich them together. Drizzle any excess chocolate on top.

Enjoy immediately!

NO-BAKE PROTEIN BROWNIE BITES

INGREDIENTS

2 oz dark chocolate bar of choice

1 tbsp Bulletproof Grass-Fed Ghee

2 scoops Bulletproof Dark Chocolate Energy Collagen Protein

¾ cup blanched almond flour

4 tbsp desiccated coconut

2 tsp vanilla extract

INSTRUCTIONS

Melt the chocolate bar and ghee in a small saucepan over medium heat.

Add all **Ingredients** to a food processor and blitz until combined.

Scrape down sides of food processor. Taste mixture, if desired, and re-blend.

In your hands, roll a bit of the mixture into a ball — it should roll easily. If too dry, blend in a touch more ghee or a small amount of water until it comes together and is easy to roll.

Roll the mixture into 14 balls and coat in extra desiccated dried coconut or (optional) toasted and finely chopped nuts or seeds.

Place on plate or in container, and refrigerate until set.

Enjoy your fudgy protein brownie bites!

PALEO PIZOOKIE – HOMEMADE SKILLET COOKIE

INGREDIENTS

1/3 cup coconut flour

2 tablespoons tapioca flour

1 scoop collagen peptides (may substitute chocolate or vanilla flavors)

1/4 teaspoon baking soda

1/4 teaspoon salt

1 teaspoon ground ceylon cinnamon

WET **INGREDIENTS**

1 pasture raised egg + 1 egg yolk

2 tablespoons Brain Octane Oil

1 1/2 tablespoons raw honey

1 teaspoon stevia

1 teaspoon vanilla extract

2/3 cup sprouted almond butter (may substitute raw almond butter, or soaked cashew nut butter)

1/2 cup dark 90% chocolate chips (may substitute cacao nibs)

Coconut oil for greasing

INSTRUCTIONS

Preheat oven to 350 degrees. Grease the base of an 8-inch cast iron skillet with coconut oil.

In a blender, add all wet **Ingredients** and blend for 1 minute. Transfer the mixture to a wide mixing bowl.

In another bowl, sieve coconut and tapioca flours. Add remaining dry **Ingredients** and mix until everything is combined.

Add dry **Ingredients** to wet **Ingredients** and stir until a dough forms. Add 3/4 of the chocolate chips and fold through.

Add pizookie dough to the skillet. Use the back of a spoon to spread the dough to the edges of the pan and smooth the top. Sprinkle remaining chocolate chips over the pizookie.

Bake for 12 minutes, or until the sides begin to puff and the top is set and starting to turn golden. Check your pizookie around the 10-minute mark, since it can overcook quickly and lose its golden color.

Remove from the oven and allow to cool for a few minutes. Serve warm with paleo or keto ice cream, or fresh organic berries.

COCONUT AND LEMON SUGAR COOKIES

INGREDIENTS

1 ¾ cups almond flour

1/4 cup coconut flour

2 tbsp Bulletproof Grass-Fed Ghee or butter, softened

1 egg

? cup granulated sweetener of your choice

1/2 tsp baking soda

1 tsp vanilla extract (substitute with half as much vanilla powder)

Pinch of salt

MCT OIL ROYAL ICING

2 tbsp Bulletproof Brain Octane C8 MCT Oil

1-1.5 tbsp powdered sweetener of choice

1/4 tsp vanilla powder (substitute with twice as much vanilla extract)

1 tbsp coconut butter (unmelted)

1 lemon , juiced

Lemon zest for garnish

INSTRUCTIONS

Mix all of the cookie **Ingredients** together until evenly combined. Roll the dough into a ball.

Cover the dough with plastic wrap and place into the fridge for 2-3 hours.

Preheat the oven to 350°F (175°C). Line a baking tray with parchment paper.

Slice the dough in half and roll one of the halves out evenly in between two pieces of parchment paper with a rolling pin. Roll into 1/4 inch thickness (or roughly 1/8 inch for thinner cookies).

Cut into shapes with cutters of your choice, or use a round drinking glass if you don't have any cookie cutters. Place cut cookies on the lined baking sheets, about 1 inch apart, then place in the freezer again for 10 minutes (to prevent spreading). Repeat this process until you've used up all of the cookie dough scraps. You should make approximately 26 cookies with this amount of dough.

Bake cookies, one sheet at a time, on the middle rack for 10-12 minutes, or until edges are light golden brown.

Remove from the oven and allow the cookies to cool on the baking sheet for about 10 minutes, or until they harden. If you've made slightly thicker cookies, the base of the cookies may still be a little blonde, so carefully turn them over and place them back into the oven to finish cooking the base until they're a light golden brown. This should take about 5 minutes, but keep an eye on them.

Once the cookies are ready, remove them from the oven and allow the cookies to cool on the baking sheet for about 15 minutes before transferring to a wire rack.

While they're cooling, you can make the icing. In a small saucepan, add all of the icing **Ingredients**and melt on a low heat. Mix until evenly combined and smooth. Taste and adjust the lemon juice or sweetener as desired.

When the cookies are completely cooled, drizzle the icing over the top of the cookies evenly and sprinkle with lemon zest. Enjoy!

CARROT CAKE COLLAGEN MUFFINS WITH CASHEW ICING

INGREDIENTS

CARROT CAKE COLLAGEN MUFFINS

1 1/2 cups blanched almond flour

1 carrot , grated (roughly 2 cups, loosely packed, per carrot)

3 eggs , beaten

? cup Bulletproof Grass-Fed Ghee , melted

? cup powdered sweetener of choice

2 tbsp tapioca flour

1 scoop Bulletproof Collagen Protein powder

2 tsp vanilla extract (substitute with half as much vanilla powder)

1.5 tsp cinnamon

1/2-1 tsp ginger powder

¾ tsp baking soda

CASHEW ICING

1 1/2 cups cashews , soaked and strained

1/4 cup coconut cream

1 tbsp Bulletproof Brain Octane C8 MCT Oil

1 tsp vanilla extract (substitute with half as much vanilla powder)

2 tbsp powdered sweetener of choice (or more to taste)

You'll only use about half the batch of Cashew Icing. Store the rest in the fridge up to a week, or freeze it for your next baking project!

INSTRUCTIONS

Preheat the oven to 350°F (175°C). Grease and line a muffin tray.

Add all the muffin **Ingredients**into a large mixing bowl and stir until evenly combined.

Scoop or pour the batter into the prepared muffin tray. Place into the oven and bake for 30-35 minutes, or until the muffins are cooked through.

Allow the muffins to cool on a wire rack while you make the Cashew Icing.

Add all of the icing **Ingredients** into a small blender or food processor. Blend until smooth. Scrape down the sides of the bowl and re-blend. Taste the icing and add a touch more sweetener or lemon juice if desired.

Pour the icing into a piping bag. Once the muffins are warm (not hot), pipe the icing on top of a muffin and enjoy!

LEMON DRIZZLE CAKE

INGREDIENTS

2 eggs

3 tbsp. Bulletproof Collagen Protein powder

1 3/4 cups almond flour

1/2 tsp. baking soda

3 tbsp. tapioca flour

Zest and juice of 2 lemons (just under 1/2 cup lemon juice)

3 tbsp. Bulletproof Grass-Fed Ghee or melted butter

1/3 cup maple syrup

COCONUT LEMON DRIZZLE ICING

1-1.5 tbsp. powdered sweetener

2 tbsp. coconut butter

2 tbsp. Bulletproof Brain Octane C8 MCT Oil

Juice of 3/4 to 1 lemon

GARNISH

Lemon zest

INSTRUCTIONS

Preheat the oven to 350°F/180°C. Grease and line a rectangular slice tin with baking paper. (I used a cake tray with these dimensions: 7.5 inch x 11 inches.)

Add all **Ingredients**into a blender and combine until smooth.

Pour into the prepared cake tin.

Place into the oven and bake for 17-20 minutes, or until the cake is cooked through.

Remove from the oven and allow to cool before icing.

Add all the Coconut Lemon Drizzle Icing **Ingredients**into a small saucepan. Melt on low until combined. Stir until completely smooth. Add more lemon juice to taste, if desired.

Place the lemon cake onto a rectangular plate or tray. Begin to drizzle the icing over the top of cake with a spoon.

Garnish with extra lemon zest. Slice and enjoy, or store in the refrigerator in an airtight container.

DELICIOUS BULLETPROOF DIET BEVERAGE RECIPES

ICED BULLETPROOF COFFEE

INGREDIENTS

1 cup Bulletproof coffee (brewed)

1 tsp Bulletproof Brain Octane C8 MCT Oil , up to 2 tbsp (see notes)

1-2 tsp Bulletproof Grass-Fed Ghee

1 cup ice to fill glass

INSTRUCTIONS

Brew 1 cup (8-12 ounces) of coffee using Bulletproof coffee beans.

Add coffee, Brain Octane C8 MCT Oil and Ghee to a blender.

Blend 20-30 seconds until it looks like a creamy latte. Allow to cool slightly.

Pour over ice. Enjoy!

BLUE SPIRULINA LATTE

INGREDIENTS

2 grams high-quality powdered blue spirulina (roughly 1/2 teaspoon)

1 tbsp Brain Octane Oil

1 tbsp coconut butter

1 heaping tablespoon collagen peptides

1 1/2 cups coconut milk

1/4 tsp ground Ceylon cinnamon

INSTRUCTIONS

In a saucepan on low heat, add coconut milk and gently warm.

While coconut milk heats up, add a small amount of the blue spirulina to a glass bowl.

When milk is warmed, add a small amount to the bowl and whisk until blue spirulina dissolves.

Keep adding more spirulina and more milk little by little. Adding too much of either at a time can cause the spirulina to clump.

After milk and spirulina are fully incorporated, add the mixture to a blender along with coconut butter, Brain Octane, and cinnamon. Blend until frothy.

Add collagen peptides and blend again on low speed until just combined to avoid damaging delicate proteins.

Pour your latte into a mug and garnish with a sprinkle of cinnamon

CARAMEL ICED COFFEE

INGREDIENTS

ICED COFFEE

3 cups almond milk, unsweetened

4 cups cold brew

3 tsp vanilla extract

3 cup ice cubes

COCONUT WHIPPED CREAM

2 cans coconut cream (full fat; refrigerate overnight)

 1/2 tbsp powdered erythritol monk fruit blend, such as Lakanto

1 tsp vanilla extract

SUGAR-FREE CARAMEL SAUCE

1 can coconut cream (full fat; refrigerate overnight)

3 tbsp Lakanto Brown Monkfruit Sweetener

2 tsp Bulletproof French Vanilla Creamer

1 tsp vanilla extract

1 pinch salt

INSTRUCTIONS

CARAMEL SAUCE

Add the coconut cream and monk fruit into a saucepan and simmer on medium heat for approximately 20-30 minutes, or until the coconut cream evaporates and thickens up. Make sure to continuously stir it after the 15-20 minute mark so it doesn't stick and burn to the bottom of the pan.

Remove from heat and whisk in salt, vanilla extract and French Vanilla Creamer. Set aside to cool while you make the whipped coconut cream.

COCONUT WHIPPED CREAM

For best results, place a small mixing bowl in the freezer for 20-30 minutes before you begin to make the whipped cream.

Open two cans of coconut milk, but be careful not to shake them! Scoop the coconut cream solids from the top of the cans into your chilled mixing bowl.

Add the sweetener and vanilla extract. Beat the mixture with a hand mixer; start on low speed to break up the coconut cream solids. If the mixture is still too thick and the coconut solid is not breaking down, add some of the liquid from the can, one teaspoon at a time. Then turn to high speed and beat for about 3-5 minutes until soft peaks form.

CARAMEL ICED COFFEE ASSEMBLY

Add all of the **Ingredients** into your blender (except ice), and blend on high for 30-60 seconds until it is smooth, creamy and frothy.

Add ice into two glasses and pour the iced coffee mixture over the top.

Pipe whipped coconut cream on top and drizzle with homemade caramel sauce.

Find a relaxing spot where you can enjoy each and every decadent sip of this keto-friendly caramel iced coffee!

KETO MOJITO RECIPE

INGREDIENTS

1.5 oz Bacardi Superior (or another Cuban-style rum)

1/2 lime (juiced)

1 scoop Vanilla Collagen Peptides

2 oz soda water

1 bunch Mint leaves

INSTRUCTIONS

Pour the rum into a tall glass, followed by lime juice and soda water.

Add Vanilla Collagen Peptides, stir well and top with crushed ice.

Clap the mint bouquet to release added aromatics before topping cocktail with fresh garnish.

Find a relaxing place to put your feet up and enjoy this keto mojito recipe, one stress-free sip at a time.

RAINBOW SMOOTHIE RECIPE

INGREDIENTS

RED LAYER

1 cup frozen strawberries

1 cup frozen raspberries

1/2 cup full-fat Greek yogurt

ORANGE LAYER

1 cup frozen oranges

1 cup frozen tangerines

1/2 cup full-fat Greek yogurt

2 scoops Unflavored Collagen Peptides*

YELLOW LAYER

2 cups frozen pineapple

1/2 cup greek yogurt

1 cup spinach

1 cup kiwi

1 cup avocado

1 tsp. Brain Octane Oil

BLUE LAYER

1 1/2 cups full-fat Greek yogurt

1/2 tsp. blue spirulina

PURPLE LAYER

2 cups frozen blueberries

1/2 cup full-fat Greek yogurt

*Add 2 scoops of Unflavored Collagen Protein to any layer, or distribute evenly between all layers

INSTRUCTIONS

Blend the **Ingredients**for each layer thoroughly. Make sure to clean your blender in between rounds.

In reverse-rainbow order, pour half the contents of each layer into a clear glass (begin with purple; end with red).

Garnish with handful of fresh herbs and berries.

Add a reusable straw and sip your rainbow smoothie to your heart's content!

KETO ICED COFFEE PROTEIN SHAKE

INGREDIENTS

 1/2 avocado (or 1/4 large avocado) frozen with skin and pit removed

4 oz Bulletproof Original Coffee brewed and frozen into cubes

1 1/4 cup unsweetened full-fat coconut milk (or milk of choice)

1 scoop Bulletproof Vanilla Collagen Peptides

1/2 tbsp Bulletproof Brain Octane C8 MCT Oil

1 tbsp cacao powder

1/4 tsp Ceylon cinnamon

1/2 cup ice (in addition to cold brew cubes)

INSTRUCTIONS

Add all **Ingredients**to a blender. Blend, starting on a low speed and working your way up.

Garnish, if desired, and serve.

PALEO FROZEN COFFEE

INGREDIENTS

2 cups ice

1 tbsp Brain Octane C8 MCT Oil

1 tbsp cacao powder

2 tsp sweetener, such as powdered stevia

4 oz Bulletproof Original Coffee brewed

INSTRUCTIONS

In a blender, add all **Ingredients**except for ice and blend until incorporated.

Add ice and blend again until mixture reaches a slushie consistency.

Pour into a glass or tumbler and enjoy!

BERRY MATCHA SMOOTHIE

INGREDIENTS

1 cup coconut milk

1 cup filtered water

1-1.5 cups frozen organic berries

 1/2 avocado

1 tbsp Bulletproof Brain Octane C8 MCT Oil

1 scoop Bulletproof Vanilla Bean Energy Collagen Protein

1 scoop Bulletproof InnerFuel Prebiotic

1 tsp matcha powder

 1/2-1 tsp vanilla extract

Optional: Ice and sweetener of choice, to taste

INSTRUCTIONS

Add all **Ingredients** into a blender and blitz until completely smooth.

Taste and adjust, as needed.

Pour into two glasses and enjoy immediately.

KETO HOT CHOCOLATE

INGREDIENTS

1 1/2 cups nut milk (we used homemade cashew milk)

1 scoop Original Creamer

2 scoops Chocolate Collagen Peptides

1/2 tsp organic cinnamon

1/2 tsp vanilla powder (substitute with twice as much vanilla extract)

Optional for mocha: Double-shot of Bulletproof Coffee

Optional for sweetness: 2-4 drops of keto-friendly liquid sweetener (like stevia or monkfruit), if desired

INSTRUCTIONS

Add all **Ingredients**into a small saucepan and warm on low heat to 160°F-170°F (70°C-80°C).

Once heated, pour into blender. Blitz on high until frothy.

Pour into two mugs, and enjoy immediately.

DELICIOUS BULLETPROOF DIET KETO RECIPES

BRUSSELS SPROUTS AU GRATIN

INGREDIENTS

2 tbsp Bulletproof Grass-Fed Ghee

1 small onion (thinly sliced)

1 lb Brussels sprouts (trimmed and quartered)

1/3 cup coconut cream

1/4 cup unsweetened almond milk

3 scoops Bulletproof Original Creamer

1 tsp salt

1/2 tsp pepper

1 tsp dried thyme

1/4 tsp nutmeg

¾ cup pork rinds (crushed)

INSTRUCTIONS

Preheat the oven to 400°F. Clean and trim the Brussels sprouts, removing the outer leaves.

Scoop the Ghee into a skillet set over medium heat. Once melted, add the sliced onions and cook for 5-8 minutes until softened.

Place the Brussels sprouts into a rectangular, 10-inch-by-7-inch baking dish (or something similar).

When the onions are done cooking, transfer them into the baking dish with the Brussels sprouts.

In the same skillet, add the coconut cream, almond milk and Creamer. Whisk until smooth.

Stir in the salt, pepper, dried thyme and nutmeg. Bring the sauce to a low simmer and cook for 2-3 minutes, stirring often.

Pour the sauce into the baking dish with the skillet and onions. Toss the vegetables with the sauce until they are evenly coated.

Transfer the dish to the oven and bake for 20 minutes.

Remove from the oven and sprinkle the crushed pork rinds on top. Return the dish to the oven and bake for another 5 minutes.

Let the Brussel sprouts au gratin cool for 5 minutes before serving.

KETO LEMON POPPY SEED MUFFINS

INGREDIENTS

MUFFIN **INGREDIENTS**

1 1/2 cups blanched almond flour

2 tbsp coconut flour

1 scoop Bulletproof Vanilla Bean Energy Collagen Protein

1/3 cup golden monk fruit-erythritol blend

1/2 tsp baking soda

1 tsp baking powder

1/4 tsp salt

1/4 cup Bulletproof Grass-Fed Ghee (melted)

3 large eggs

1/2 tsp vanilla extract

1 1/2 tbsp lemon zest

1/4 cup fresh lemon juice

2 tbsp unsweetened almond milk

1 1/2 tbsp poppy seeds

GLAZE INGREDIENTS

1/3 cup powdered monk fruit-erythritol blend

1 tbsp unsweetened almond milk

1/4 tsp vanilla extract

1-2 tsp fresh lemon juice

INSTRUCTIONS

Preheat the oven to 425°F. Line a muffin tin with baking cups.

In a large mixing bowl, combine the almond flour, coconut flour, Vanilla Bean Energy Collagen Protein, monk fruit sweetener, baking soda, baking powder and salt. Whisk together to remove any lumps in the dry ingredients. Create a well in the center.

Pour the melted Grass-Fed Ghee into the dry-ingredient well. Add the eggs, vanilla, lemon zest, lemon juice and almond milk. Stir the wet

Ingredientstogether, slowly incorporating the dry ingredients. Mix until combined.

Stir in the poppy seeds.

Spoon the batter into the muffin cups, filling each one ¾ of the way full.

Transfer to the center rack of the oven and bake for 5 minutes at 425°F, then lower the oven temperature to 350°F and continue baking for 15-17 minutes, or until the muffins are a light golden-brown on top. If the muffins start to brown too quickly, place a sheet of parchment paper on top.

Remove from the oven and cool for 5 minutes in the muffin pan. Transfer each muffin to a cooling rack to cool completely.

Next, make the glaze. Mix the powdered sweetener, almond milk and vanilla extract in a small bowl. Whisk in 1 teaspoon of lemon juice. Taste and add more lemon juice as needed.

Dip each muffin into the glaze, swirling around to cover the muffin tops completely. Allow any excess glaze to drip off, then place the muffin on a plate or baking rack to let the glaze set.

Enjoy these keto lemon poppy seed muffins with a cup of clean, toxin-tested coffee for the ultimate food-and-coffee pairing.

NO-BAKE KETO CHOCOLATE CHIP COOKIES

INGREDIENTS

1/3 cup Bulletproof Grass-Fed Ghee (melted)

1/4 cup almond butter

3 scoops Bulletproof Vanilla Collagen Peptides

1 1/4 cups blanched almond flour

1/2 Keto-friendly chocolate bar (chopped)

1/4 tsp salt

INSTRUCTIONS

In a medium mixing bowl, whisk together the melted Ghee and almond butter until well combined.

Add the Vanilla Collagen Peptides, almond flour and salt. Mix well to form a thick cookie dough consistency.

Stir in the chopped chocolate bar. After mixing in the chopped chocolate, taste the dough and add more chocolate if desired.

Line a small baking sheet or large plate with parchment paper. Using a cookie dough scoop, spoon portions of the dough onto the parchment paper. Gently pat each cookie to slightly flatten.

Place the cookies in the freezer for at least 30 minutes to set, then enjoy chilled. Store remaining cookies in the refrigerator or the freezer.

NOTES

To freeze, transfer the cookies to a freezer-safe, airtight container lined with parchment paper. Store them in the freezer for up to 1 month.

SPIKED VANILLA MOCHA LATTE

INGREDIENTS

1 scoop Bulletproof French Vanilla Creamer

1 Bulletproof The Original Espresso Pod (freshly brewed)

2 oz bourbon

6 oz cashew milk (warmed)

2 tbsp whipped coconut cream (or sugar-free whipped cream)

1 square Bulletproof Sea Salt Dark Chocolate Bar (zested)

INSTRUCTIONS

Brew the espresso and warm the cashew milk.

Pour the cashew milk into a glass mug, followed by the espresso.

Add the scoop of Creamer and froth until combined for 30 seconds.

Top with the bourbon.

Finish with sugar-free whipped cream, followed by garnishing with a freshly zested Chocolate Bar.

PUMPKIN PIE FAT BOMBS

INGREDIENTS

2 tbsp Bulletproof MCT Oil

2 scoops Bulletproof Vanilla Bean Energy Collagen Protein

1/2 cup coconut butter

1/4 cup coconut oil (extra virgin)

2 tsp pumpkin pie spice

1 tbsp Lakanto Powdered Monkfruit Sweetener (or powdered low-carb sweetener of choice)

1/2 cup unsweetened pumpkin puree

1 tsp vanilla extract (or powder)

INSTRUCTIONS

Place the coconut butter, coconut oil, powdered sweetener, vanilla and pumpkin spice mix into a small saucepan and melt to combine over a low-medium heat.

Add the pumpkin puree and mix until well combined.

Remove from the heat once combined. Stir in the collagen protein powder thoroughly to make sure there are no lumps.

Add a heaping teaspoon of the mixture into every mini muffin cup. Place into the fridge and let it set.

When done, keep refrigerated in an airtight container, as the coconut oil and butter get very soft at room temperature

EASY SEARED STEAK WITH GHEE

INGREDIENTS

10 ounces Crowd Cow grass-fed, grass finished New York Strip Steak

2 tbsp Bulletproof Grass-Fed Ghee

Salt and pepper to taste

Brain Octane Oil to finish (optional)

INSTRUCTIONS

Heat a cast-iron skillet over medium-high heat and add Grass-Fed Ghee to melt. While your skillet heats, pat the steak dry and liberally season with salt and pepper on both sides.

Once the ghee melts and the skillet is hot, add the steak to the skillet and cook on both sides until golden brown and cooked to your liking, about 2-3 minutes per side for medium rare, flipping once.

Remove steak from the pan and let rest for 10 minutes.

Slice the steak and finish with a drizzle of Brain Octane oil.

PUMPKIN SPICE KETO GRANOLA RECIPE

INGREDIENTS

1 cup sunflower seeds

1 cup pumpkin seeds

1 cup pecans

1 cup almonds (chopped)

1 cup cashews (chopped)

1/2 cup Brazil nuts (chopped)

2 cups coconut flakes (unsweetened)

3 tbsp granulated sweetener, such as non-GMO erythritol or birch xylitol

3 tbsp Bulletproof Grass-Fed Ghee

2 tbsp Bulletproof Brain Octane C8 MCT Oil

1 scoop Bulletproof Unflavored Collagen Protein

1-2 tsp vanilla extract

1 tbsp pumpkin pie spice

INSTRUCTIONS

Preheat oven to 320ºF. Line a large baking tray with parchment paper.

Add all **Ingredients**into a large bowl (except for the collagen powder) and mix until everything is evenly coated.

Pour onto the lined baking sheet evenly, place into the oven and bake for 15 minutes.

Remove tray from oven, toss the mixture so all sides get evenly toasted and place back into oven to bake for another 7-10 minutes, or until golden brown. NOTE: Be sure to keep an eye on it so your keto granola recipe doesn't burn!

Remove from oven and stir in the collagen protein powder while the granola is still warm.

Allow to cool completely before transferring to a large glass jar or airtight container to store at room temperature.

For a quick keto breakfast, serve in a bowl with your milk of choice, atop a heap of probiotic coconut yogurt and berries, or for added crunch to your morning smoothie bowl.

CARAMEL ICED COFFEE

INGREDIENTS

ICED COFFEE

3 cups almond milk, unsweetened

4 cups cold brew

3 tsp vanilla extract

3 cup ice cubes

COCONUT WHIPPED CREAM

2 cans coconut cream (full fat; refrigerate overnight)

1/2 tbsp powdered erythritol monk fruit blend, such as Lakanto

1 tsp vanilla extract

SUGAR-FREE CARAMEL SAUCE

1 can coconut cream (full fat; refrigerate overnight)

3 tbsp Lakanto Brown Monkfruit Sweetener

2 tsp Bulletproof French Vanilla Creamer

1 tsp vanilla extract

1 pinch salt

INSTRUCTIONS

CARAMEL SAUCE

Add the coconut cream and monk fruit into a saucepan and simmer on medium heat for approximately 20-30 minutes, or until the coconut cream evaporates and thickens up. Make sure to continuously stir it after the 15-20 minute mark so it doesn't stick and burn to the bottom of the pan.

Remove from heat and whisk in salt, vanilla extract and French Vanilla Creamer. Set aside to cool while you make the whipped coconut cream.

COCONUT WHIPPED CREAM

For best results, place a small mixing bowl in the freezer for 20-30 minutes before you begin to make the whipped cream.

Open two cans of coconut milk, but be careful not to shake them! Scoop the coconut cream solids from the top of the cans into your chilled mixing bowl.

Add the sweetener and vanilla extract. Beat the mixture with a hand mixer; start on low speed to break up the coconut cream solids. If the mixture is still too thick and the coconut solid is not breaking down, add some of the liquid from the can, one teaspoon at a time. Then turn to high speed and beat for about 3-5 minutes until soft peaks form.

CARAMEL ICED COFFEE ASSEMBLY

Add all of the **Ingredients**into your blender (except ice), and blend on high for 30-60 seconds until it is smooth, creamy and frothy.

Add ice into two glasses and pour the iced coffee mixture over the top.

Pipe whipped coconut cream on top and drizzle with homemade caramel sauce.

Find a relaxing spot where you can enjoy each and every decadent sip of this keto-friendly caramel iced coffee

COBB SALAD SKEWERS

INGREDIENTS

SALAD

6 butter lettuce leaves

5 hard-boiled eggs (halved or quartered)

1 avocado (peeled and sliced into chunks)

8 strips bacon

10 cherry tomatoes

1/2 lemon, juiced

10 bamboo skewers

DRESSING

5 tbsp balsamic vinegar

1-2 tbsp Bulletproof Brain Octane C8 MCT Oil

INSTRUCTIONS

Add the chopped avocado into a small bowl and cover it in the lemon juice evenly. This will help prevent the avocado from browning.

Slice the lettuce leaves into bite-sized square pieces.

Fold the bacon into bite-sized pieces.

Begin to layer the salad onto the skewers in any order. (Note: We made approximately 10.)

Add the balsamic vinegar and Brain Octane MCT Oil into a small dish and stir to combine.

Place the skewers onto a serving dish and drizzle with dressing.

Hand out your cobb salad skewers to friends and family, and enjoy!

BULLETPROOF GUACAMOLE WITHBRAIN OCTANE MCT OIL

INGREDIENTS

4 large ripe Haas avocados

2-4 tbsp Brain Octane MCT oil

2 tsp or more of Himalayan salt (to taste)

1 tbsp dried oregano

1-3 tsp apple cider vinegar (to taste)

Optional add-ins: chopped cilantro, jalapeños

INSTRUCTIONS

Blend everything with a hand blender until it is very creamy.

Stir in chopped cilantro and jalapeños (if you tolerate nightshades) or other herbs of your choice.

Enjoy on top of grass fed meat, sushi, salads or pretty much anything.

PART FIVE: Biohacking Your Lifestyle

Using the Bulletproof Diet as a guide, you may biohack your lifestyle in order to improve your health, performance, and overall happiness. Sleep, stress, exercise, and cognitive performance are all part of this approach's daily coverage. Some examples of lifestyle biohacks include making sure you get enough sleep each night by sticking to a regular schedule, making sure your bedroom is cool, dark, and quiet, and utilizing tools like a weighted blanket or glasses that block blue light to help you drift off to dreamland. Mindfulness meditation, deep breathing techniques, and yoga are some biohacks for stress management that can help lower cortisol levels and increase relaxation.

Improve your cardiovascular health, muscular strength, and endurance using exercise biohacks like high-intensity interval training (HIIT), resistance training, or low-impact sports like swimming or walking. Brain training activities or puzzles may test cognitive ability, and nutrients like omega-3 fatty acids or adaptogenic herbs can help keep the brain healthy and clear of fog. These are all examples of cognitive function biohacks. Enhance your overall health and performance by adding these lifestyle biohacks into your everyday routine. They work hand in hand with the Bulletproof Diet principles for best results.

Sleep Optimization and Stress Management

As part of the Bulletproof Diet, you may optimize your sleep by following certain steps to increase the amount and quality of your slumber, which is crucial to your health. If you want to improve your sleep quality using biohacks, some things you can do include sticking to a regular sleep schedule, making sure your bedroom is cold and dark, and developing a soothing ritual just before bed. Meditation and deep breathing exercises are two more relaxation strategies that can help you get a good night's sleep by calming your mind and body. To improve the quality of sleep and reduce the negative impact of artificial light on melatonin generation, you can use blue light-blocking glasses or applications that change the brightness of your screen.

Because of the detrimental effects that stress may have on health and performance, stress management is a cornerstone of the Bulletproof

Diet way of life. Some examples of biohacks for stress management include making time each day for mindfulness techniques like yoga or meditation to help you unwind and lower your cortisol levels. Exercising regularly, whether it's strength training or cardiovascular exercise, releases endorphins and boosts mood, both of which can help reduce stress. To further aid with stress management, making time for leisure activities, being outdoors, and building social relationships should all be priorities.

When it comes to Bulletproof Diet health and performance optimization, mobility and exercise are king. One example of a biohack for movement and exercise is to mix up your workouts. Try jogging or cycling for cardio, strength training using your own body weight or resistance bands, and yoga or Pilates for flexibility. The detrimental impacts of sitting for extended periods can be mitigated and general physical health and vitality can be enhanced by interspersing small periods of activity throughout the day, such as stretching or going for a walk. Individuals may improve their general health and support the Bulletproof Diet's principles for peak performance and wellness by making these sleep optimization, stress management, and exercise habits a regular part of their lives.